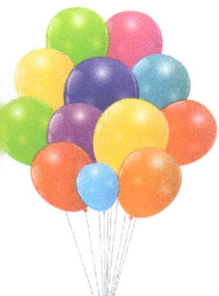

Welcome to Our Practice

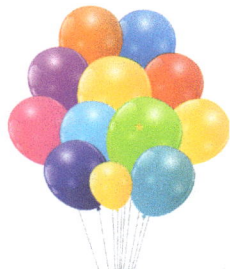

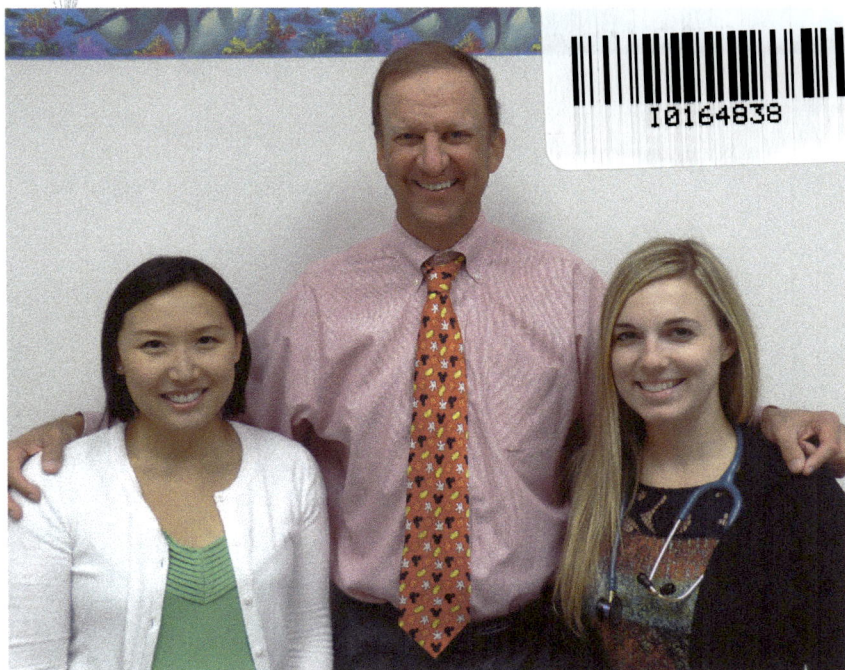

Children's Care Pediatrics

At Children's Care Pediatrics, we strive to provide excellent care for your children in a professional and courteous manner. We pride ourselves in maintaining a friendly and relaxed environment. We take the time necessary to take great care of your child and make sure all your questions are answered.

CHILDREN'S CARE PEDIATRICS

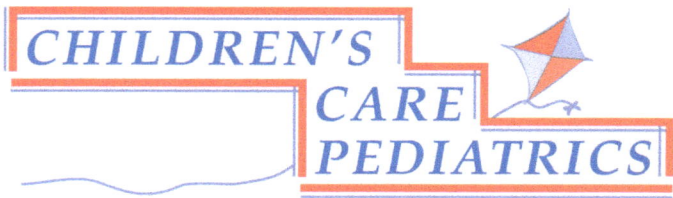

Putting CARE back in HealthCare

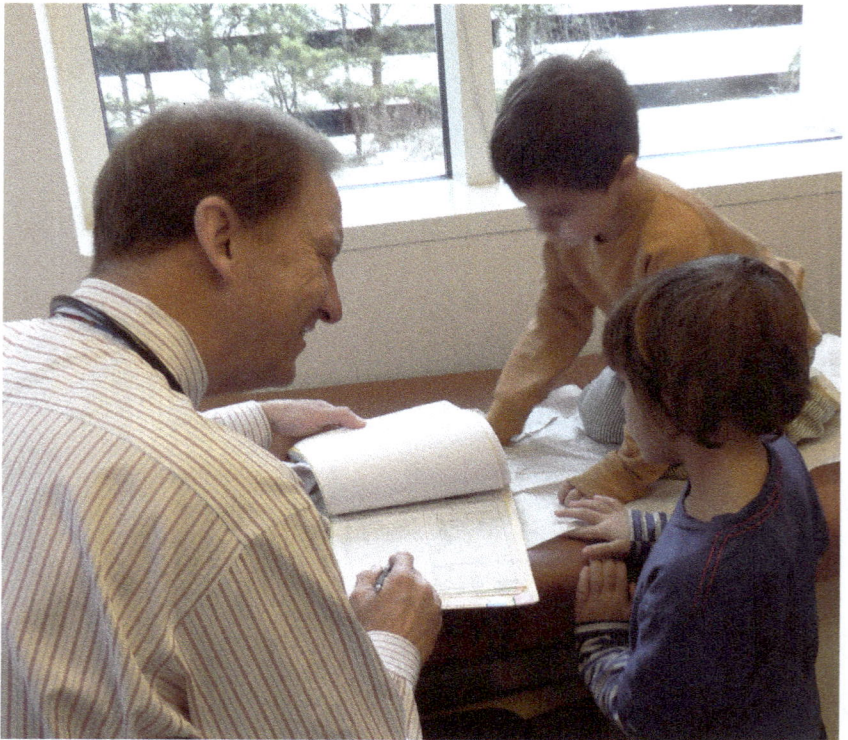

Caring For Your Baby © 2015 by Dr. John Thomas and Children's Care Pediatrics.
Published © 2015 by Overlook Connection Press, PO Box 1934, Hiram, Georgia 30141
overlookcn@aol.com
First Paperback edition ISBN: 978-1-62330-070-8

Welcome

Congratulations on your new bundle of joy! Thank you for choosing our practice to care for your child. Please use this booklet as a resource for any questions and concerns that may arise.

– The Providers & Staff at Children's Care Pediatrics

Office Hours

We have established convenient office hours to accommodate most working schedules.

Office Number: **404-705-3100**

Office Hours: Monday, Wednesday, Thursday and Friday 8:00 a.m. – 5:00 p.m.

Tuesday 9:00 a.m. – 5:00 p.m.

Saturday 9:00 a.m. for sick visits

After Hours

We ask you that you call the office during normal office hours for routine questions or non urgent illnesses. If your child should have an urgent issue that cannot wait until office hours, call the office number and a nurse or doctor will return your call within one (1) hour.

Emergencies

If you are experiencing an emergency, please call 911 or visit your nearest emergency room – whichever is most appropriate.

Child's Name:_____

Date of Birth:_____ Time:_____

Birth Weight:_____ Length:_____

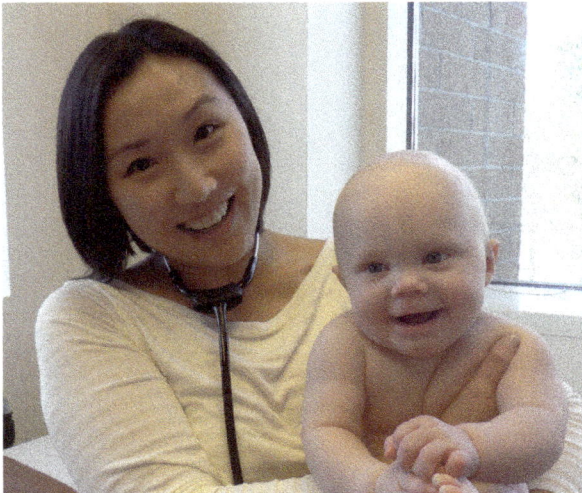

Umbilical Cord Care

Part of the umbilical cord will stay attached to your baby and will fall off usually between 1 to 4 weeks. When the cord is separating, it's normal for your baby to have a little yellow drainage or a small amount of blood for a few days. It's important to keep the umbilical cord dry. Exposing the cord to air will help with the drying process. Fold the front of your baby's diaper down so it does not cover the cord and get wet with urine. Only give your baby sponge baths until the cord falls off. It's important for the cord to fall off on its own. Even if it's hanging on by a thread, do not pull off the cord.

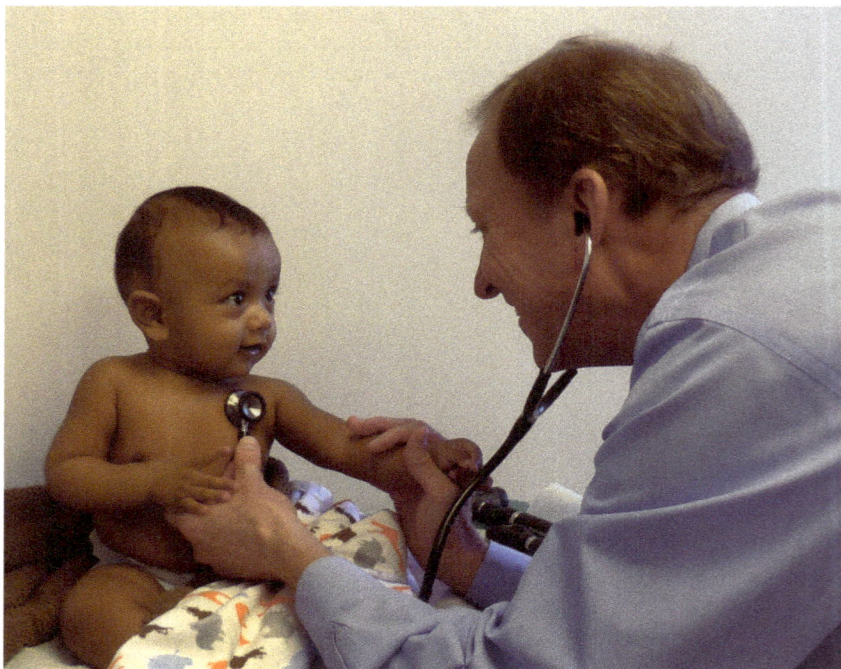

Jaundice

Jaundice is a common condition in newborns. It is a yellow discoloration in a newborn baby's skin and eyes caused by excess bilirubin in the blood. Bilirubin is produced by the normal breakdown of red blood cells. Often, treatment is not necessary, and in cases where treatment is needed usually a light therapy is used.

Bowel Movements & Constipation

Your baby's first bowel movements will be a thick black or dark-green substance called meconium. Meconium filled your baby's intestines before birth. Once all the meconium has passed, the stools will turn to a yellow-green color. Breastfed babies will have stools that resemble light mustard with seedlike particles and a consistency ranging from very soft to loose and runny. Formula-fed babies usually have bowel movements less frequently. Stool is more solid and can be a variety of colors including tan, green or yellow. Some babies will have 8 stools a day and some may only have a bowel movement every 4 days. This is not a cause for concern. If your baby is not making wet diapers (urinating 4 times over 24 hours) or not having messy diapers (stools) once a day in the first few days of life, it may be a sign that your baby is not eating well so please call the office right away.

Many parents are concerned their baby is constipated when they turn red and appear to be straining while passing stool. This is very normal, as long as the stool is normal, your baby has an appetite and the stool is not hard.

Your baby is experiencing constipation if his stools are very hard or he is not producing stool, causing him to not eat and be in discomfort. Please call our office if your baby is experiencing constipation.

Hiccups

It's very common for babies to get hiccups. This is more bothersome to you than your child. If your child gets the hiccups during a feeding, change his position or try to burp him. Stop feeding until the hiccups are gone. If the hiccups have not gone away within 5 to 10 minutes, try feeding again. This will often help them go away. Feeding your baby before he gets very hungry can often help prevent hiccups during a feeding.

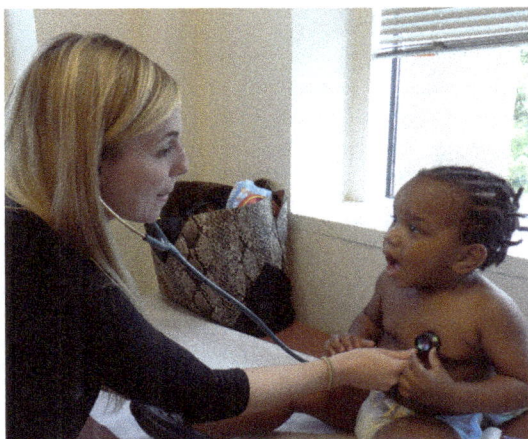

Eye Drainage

During the newborn period, eye drainage can occur, most likely due to a blocked tear duct. In newborns, tears are produced on the outside corner of the eye and then move towards the nose to drain. Since a baby's tear duct is very small, it can easily be clogged due to mucus, causing the eye to drain. If this happens, massage the inner corner of the eye and gently wipe the mucus away with a cloth or cotton ball. If drainage continues or the eye becomes red, please call our office.

Colic & Crying

Babies cry for many reasons – they are hungry, wet, too hot, too cold, tired, sick, want attention, etc. You will begin to notice the difference between the cries and what your baby wants. Crying is their only way of communicating at this early age. Don't worry about giving your baby too much attention – when he is really young, pick him up and cuddle him when he is crying.

If you are feeling overwhelmed by your crying baby, take some time away from your baby. This is a normal feeling. Ask a family member or friend to come watch your baby so you can step out for a walk. Or, if he is fed, burped and changed, place him in his crib for 10 to 15 minutes and step out of the room. **Remember to NEVER shake your baby.** Many babies become fussy around 6 p.m. – often the same time their parents arrive home from work.

Female Genitalia

Due to the mother's hormones, your baby's vagina and vulva may have some reactions which are very normal. The labia may be red and swollen, lasting just the first month. She may also have a whitish vaginal discharge or occasionally a bloody discharge. The discharge is a result of hormones present at birth, it will resolve over 1 month.

Male Genitalia

Uncircumcised Penis

In the first few months of life, you should clean your son's penis with soap and warm water like the rest of his body. Do not try to pull back the skin as it is connected by tissue to the head of the penis. Retracting the foreskin is not necessary.

Circumcised Penis

If you choose to have your son circumcised, it is most often done on the second or third day after birth. After the circumcision, at every diaper change, place a piece of gauze with petroleum jelly over the penis then put on the new diaper.

Keeping this area clean while it heals is very important – clean the area with warm soapy water if any stool gets on the penis.

You may see some redness and/or yellow secretion at the tip of the penis. This is very normal. The area should heal within a week of the procedure.

Teeth

Babies often begin teething between 3 to 6 months. Common signs for teething are drooling, chewing on objects and crankiness. To help soothe the pain, use a teething ring or Orajel®. Do not put the teething ring in a freezer.

You can also give your baby over-the-counter medications such as TYLENOL®.

Age	Recommended Dental Care
< 1 Year	Wipe your baby's teeth and gums with a wet cloth to remove any food.
1 – 2 Years	Use a soft infant toothbrush with water or infant toothpaste. It is best to brush after breakfast and before bedtime. Limit the amount of juice your child drinks to help prevent tooth problems.
2 – 3 Years	Your toddler should brush twice a day with a child-sized soft toothbrush and toothpaste. Encourage your child to brush on his own, but you should brush them again when he is done to make sure he got a good cleaning. Take your child to the dentist for a cleaning at least once a year.
> 3 Years	Your child should continue brushing twice a day and should have two cleanings a year from the dentist.

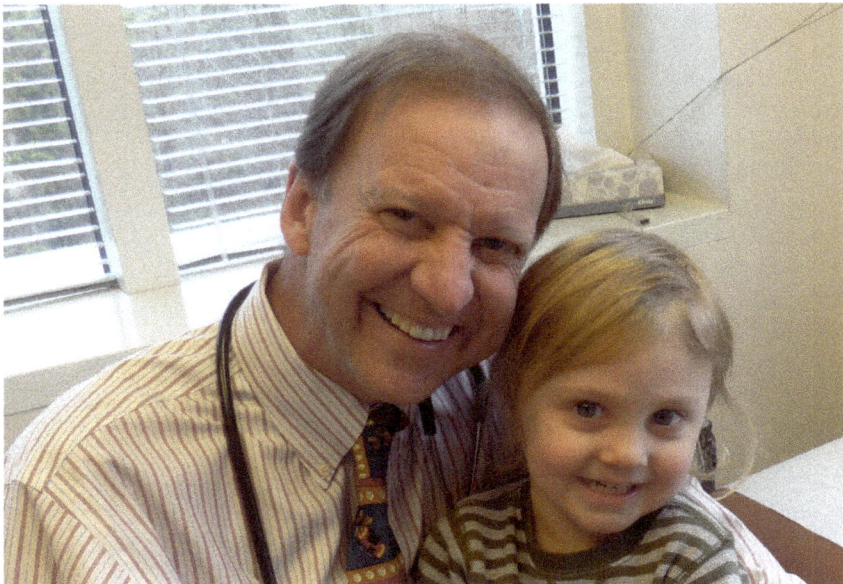

Feeding

Feeding Time

Feeding time is your baby's favorite time. Both you and your baby should enjoy the closeness that feeding time brings. Your baby should be dry and warm before starting a feeding. Babies should be fed every 3 to 4 hours during the day, but at night allow your baby to sleep as long as he wants.

Sterilization

Sterilizing your bottles is not always necessary. A dishwasher or hot soapy water washing will work just fine.

Burping

Babies often get fussy when they swallow a lot of air. Both breastfed and bottle-fed babies will swallow air during feedings, but it is more common in bottle-fed babies. If your baby begins to fuss while feeding, it's best to stop feeding and burp him. When feeding, you should burp frequently to decrease the amount of air he takes in. A breastfed baby, should be burped between breasts and a bottle-fed baby should be burped every 2 to 3 ounces. Burping after a feeding and holding your baby upright for 20-30 minutes after a feeding can help with spit up and reflux symptoms.

Formula Feeding

Every baby is different and their feedings are unique. Over time you will figure out your baby's schedule and needs. After the first few days of life, a formula-fed baby may take about 2 to 3 ounces every three to four hours for the first few weeks. By the end of the first month, some babies will be up to 4 ounces a feeding. Between 2 to 4 months, some babies will be eating enough that he no longer needs a feeding in the middle of the night. At 6 months of age, he will be eating four to five times a day at 6 to 8 ounces per feeding. Your baby will reach a maximum of 7 to 8 ounces per feeding. He should not drink more than 32 ounces of formula in a 24-hour period.

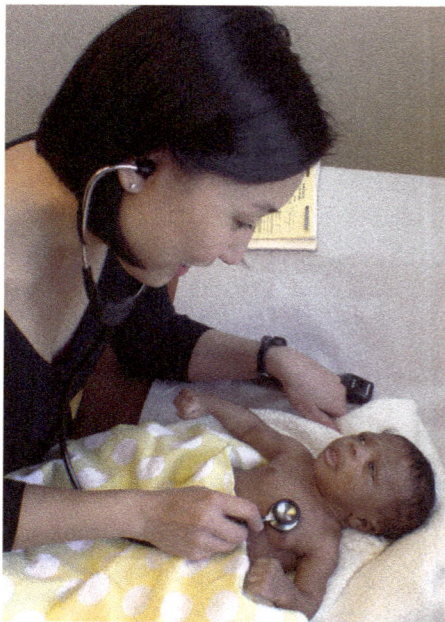

Breastfeeding

Breastfeeding does not always come easy. Be patient and confident that you can breastfeed your baby. It is often uncomfortable for the first few weeks until you and your baby learn to latch properly. During the first few weeks, your baby will feed 8 to 12 times a day. If you're having trouble getting your baby alert to latch on, undress him down to a diaper and place him against your bare chest. You will begin to notice when your baby wants to eat – watch for rooting, licking and sucking. If you wait for your child to cry, you may have a harder time getting a good latch. Typically your baby will nurse 10 to 15 minutes on each side.

Breast & Nipple Care

Breastfeeding can be tough on your breasts and nipples. The following tips will help keep your breasts and nipples healthy, making breastfeeding more enjoyable.

- When bathing, wash and dry breasts and nipples as you normally would.
- While bathing, massage your breast and soften out any hard spots you may find.
- If you leak milk onto breast pads, change them to keep the nipple dry and rash-free.
- Wear a soft and supportive bra without underwires. Underwires can sometimes block milk flow.
- After feeding, leave a little expressed milk on the nipple and let it air dry.
- Apply lanolin cream frequently if your nipples are dry, cracked or bleeding

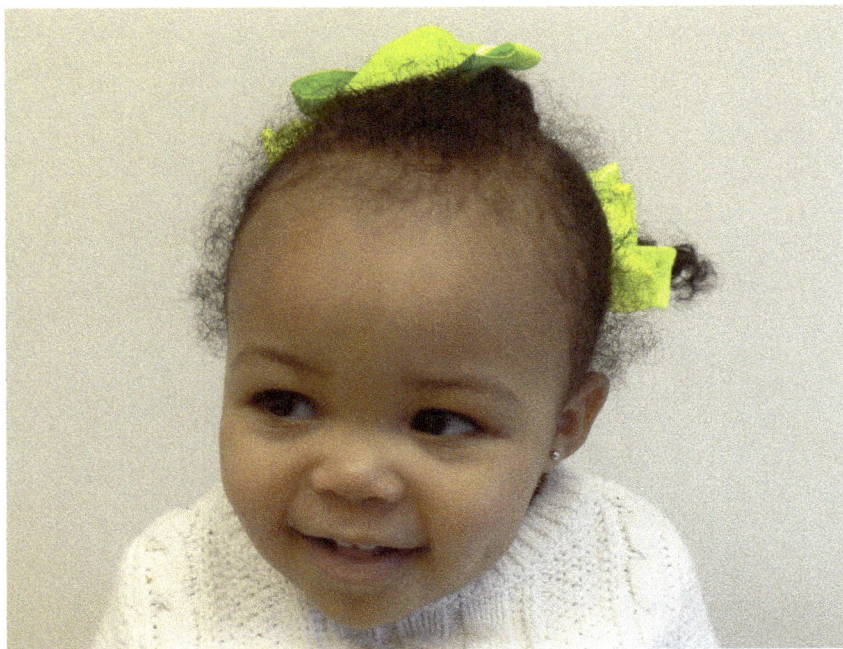

Breastmilk Storage

	Freshly Expressed Breastmilk	Thawed Breastmilk (Previously Frozen)
Room Temperature	6-8 Hours up to 77°F	Do Not Store
Insulated Cooler Bag with Frozen Ice Packs	24 Hours at 5-39°F	Do Not Store
Refrigerator	5 Days at 32-39°F	24 Hours
Self-contained Refrigerator Freezer Unit	3-6 Months at 0°F	Never Refreeze Thawed Milk
Deep Freezer	6-12 Months at -4°F	Never Refreeze Thawed Milk

Storing Breastmilk Tips

- Wash your hands before expressing or handling any milk.
- Store your breastmilk in screw-cap bottles or bags specifically designed for breastmilk.
- Freeze your milk if you do not plan to use it within 24 hours. Store it in the back where it is the coldest and away from the door, but do not put it against the wall of the freezer.
- Label all your breastmilk with the date and time it was expressed and use your oldest milk first. If giving it to a caregiver, clearly label it with your child's name.
- Freeze milk in 2 to 5 oz portions to reduce the amount of waste.
- Do not add fresh milk to already frozen milk.
- Thaw your milk in the refrigerator or by placing it in a warm bowl of water.
- If your baby does not finish all his milk during a feeding, do not save that milk for a future feeding – discard it.

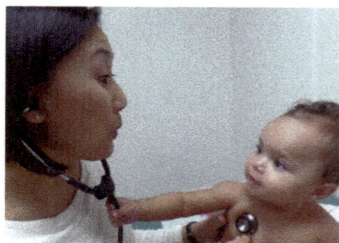

Spitting Up

Spitting up is very common with infants. This most often occurs when your baby eats more than his stomach can handle, or he burps or drools. Some babies spit up more than others. The good news is they usually outgrow it by the time they can sit up. Spitting up can be messy, but don't be concerned. It is very normal and almost never is a danger to your child. It's important to know the difference between spitting up and vomiting. When your child vomits, it will be forceful and cause discomfort. If your baby vomits frequently, you should contact our office.

Spitting up can occur no matter what you do, but below are a few tips to help manage spit up.

1. Feed your baby in a calm and quiet environment.

2. Avoid interruptions, sudden noises, bright lights, and other distractions during feedings.

3. Burp a bottlefed baby at least every 3 to 5 minutes during feedings.

4. Do not feed your baby while he is laying down.

5. Hold your baby upright for 20 to 30 minutes after each feeding.

6. Do not play or move your baby around alot right after a feeding.

7. Try to feed your baby before he gets frantically hungry.

8. When bottle feeding, make sure the hole in the nipple is the correct size. If it is too large, the formula will flow too fast, and if it is too small your baby will get frustrated and gulp for air. To see if you have the right size, invert the bottle and then stop. A few drops should come out.

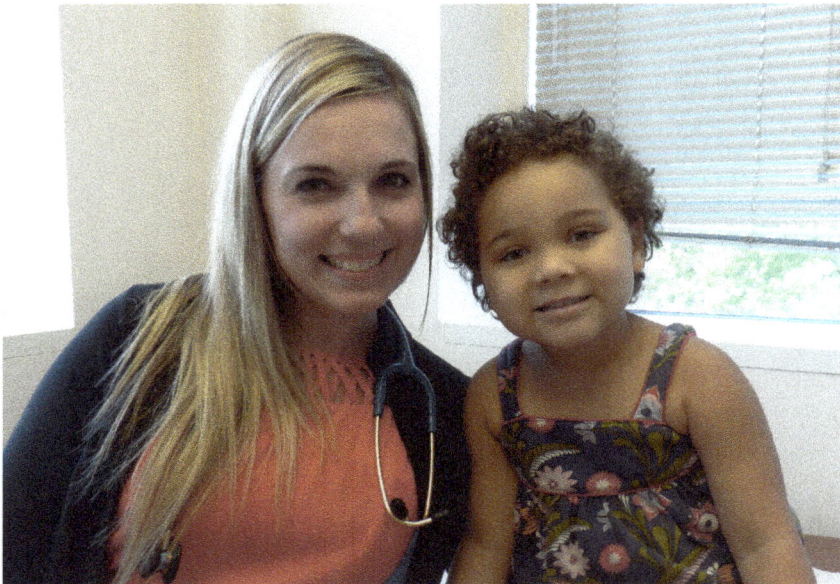

Bathing & Skin Care

Bathing

After your baby is born, you will sponge bathe him only with a warm, damp washcloth until the umbilical cord has fallen off. A regular bath can be given once the umbilical cord has fallen off and in the case for circumcised boys, the circumcision has healed. A baby should have a bath every day. Applying a baby unscented cream after a bath can help prevent dry skin.

Before bathing your child, it's important to be fully prepared. If you forgot something, the phone rings or someone is at the door, take your baby with you or ignore it – **NEVER leave your baby unattended in the tub, even for a second.**

Diaper Rash

Diaper rashes are very common in babies and are most commonly caused by his urination, bowel movements or sweat. When your baby has a diaper rash, wash his diaper area after each change with warm water. Soaps and baby wipes can cause irritation. It's important to try and keep the area as dry as possible. This includes keeping him out of a diaper as much as possible. After changing his dirty diaper, lay him on a towel allowing the diaper area to breathe. Also, use a diaper ointment containing zinc oxide, such as Desitin or A&D ointment, with each diaper change.

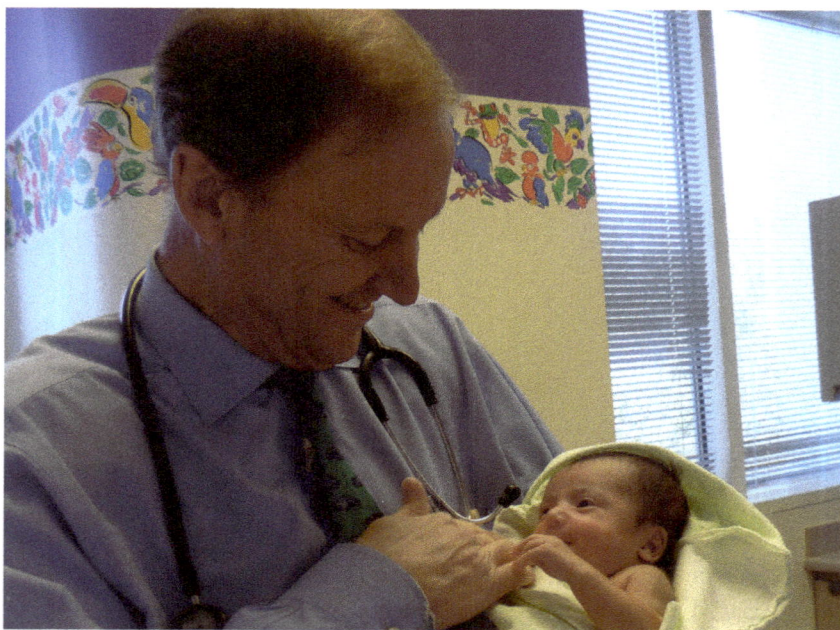

Cradle Cap

Cradle cap causes thick and crusty, white or yellow scales on your baby's scalp. Some children only have a small patch, whereas others may have scales all over their head. Cradle cap can even occur on the eyebrows, eyelids, ears, crease of the nose, back of the neck, diaper area, or armpits. Cradle cap usually resolves itself in a few months. To help clear it up, you can wash your baby's hair with a mild soap – helping to loosen up the scales. For severe conditions, make an appointment to have your baby seen.

Milia & Baby Acne

Milia are little white bumps on the nose, chin or cheeks. Most babies are born with it. It is caused by trapped skin flakes near the surface of the skin. Baby acne is more defined and appears as red or white bumps on the baby's face. Baby acne develops within the first month of life due to hormonal changes. Both milia and baby acne will clear up on their own. All you should do is wash your baby's face with water and a mild soap daily, avoid lotions and oils, and never pinch or scrub the bumps.

Nail Care

Your baby's fingernails and toenails are very soft; however, they grow very quickly. To prevent your baby from scratching his face and eyes, they should be filed or trimmed. If you clip your baby's nails, it's important to cut them straight across so you don't cut the skin which can cause an infection. It may be easier to trim your baby's nails while he is sleeping. The first 3 weeks the nails may by soft and difficult to trim so it may be easier to file them. They may have to be filed every 1-2 days.

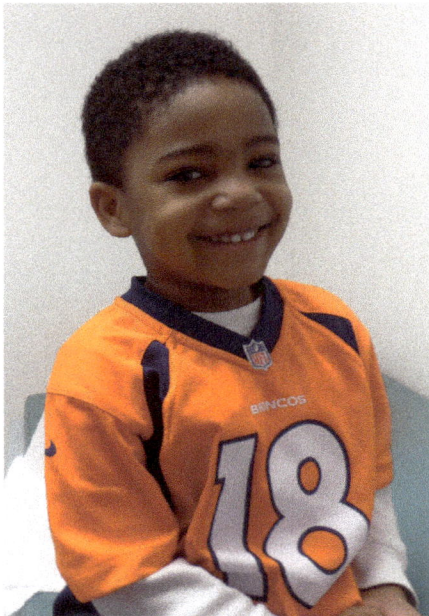

Sleeping

Infant Sleeping

Babies do not have regular sleep cycles until at least 6 months of age. As babies get older, they need less sleep. Every baby is different and has different needs for sleeping.

Always put your baby on his back to sleep to reduce the risk of Sudden Infant Death Syndrome (SIDS). SIDS is the leading cause of death for infants between the ages of 1 and 12 months.

Sleep Chart

Age	Nighttime Sleep (Hrs)	Daytime Sleep (Hrs)	No. of Naps	Total Sleep (Hrs)
1 Month	8	8	(Inconsistent)	16
3 Months	10	5	3	15
6 Months	11	3.25	2	14.25
9 Months	11	3	2	14
12 Months	11.25	2.5	2	13.75
18 Months	11.25	2.25	1	13.5
2 Years	11	2	1	13
3 Years	10.5	1.5	1	12

Crib Safety

Your baby's crib should be completely empty – this includes no pillows, blankets, toys, etc. When choosing a crib, make sure it meets all the current safety guidelines. Antique and used cribs may appear to be nice, but they may not be safe. Never use a crib with drop rails. Crib bumpers should also not be used in your baby's crib. They pose a risk of suffocation, strangulation or entrapment. Also, once your baby is older, he can use them for climbing out of the crib.

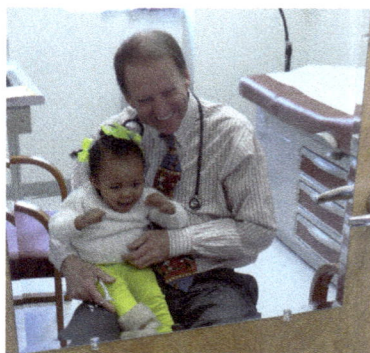

Swaddling

Research shows that swaddling your baby will help keep him calm and sleep longer because swaddling mimics the warm coziness of his mother's womb. It is important that when swaddling, you do it properly so it is snug around your baby and would never come loose – but not too tight. Also, only swaddle your baby when it is time to sleep because a swaddled baby will often sleep longer and not wake as easily. To reduce the risk of SIDS, your baby should always be put on his back to sleep. Stop swaddling your baby by 2 months of age, or once he begins to start trying to roll over.

How to Swaddle

- Spread the blanket flat, with one corner folded down.
- Lay your baby face-up on the blanket, placing his head at the edge of the folded corner.
- Straighten his left arm, and wrap the left corner of the blanket over his body and tuck it between his right arm and the right side of his body.
- Fold the bottom point of the blanket up, leaving room for his feet to move freely.
- Tuck the right arm down, and fold the right corner of the blanket over his body and under his left side.
- Make sure his hips can move and that the blanket is not too tight. You should be able to get at least two or three fingers between the baby's chest and the swaddle.

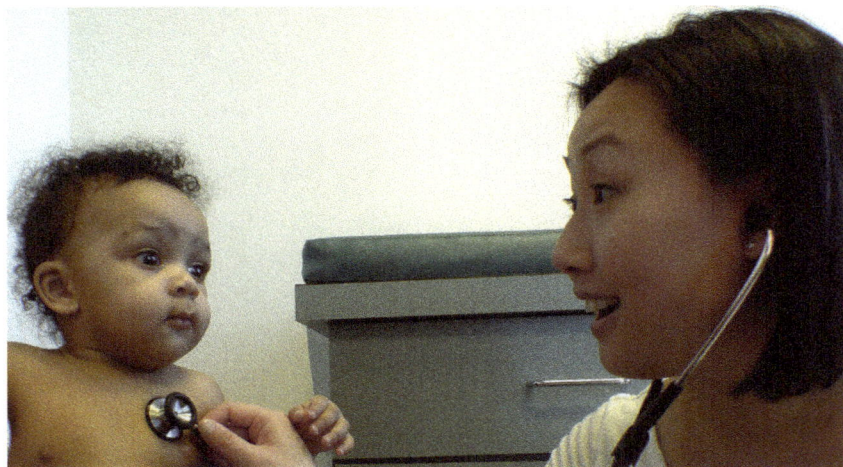

Illness

Cold & Cough

A cold is a very common illness in children. Most children will average 8 to 10 colds in their first two years of life. If your child has older siblings or is in daycare, he may have more. Colds are easily passed between children who are in close contact to each other. The cold will most likely start with a clear runny nose, then turning into a yellow or greenish discharge. Other symptoms include sneezing, low fever, decrease in appetite, fussiness and mild cough. A typical cold will resolve itself in 7 days. If the symptoms worsen or your child is under the age of 3 months, call our office for an appointment.

There are a few at home treatments you can give your child to help treat a cold.

- **Nasal Drops** – If your child has thick mucus, use saline nasal drops to help clear the nostril. Also use a nasal aspirator to help clear the mucus.

- **Fluids** – Your child should drink plenty of fluids. Even if your child doesn't have an appetite, continue to offer a drink.

- **Sit up** – Have your baby sit in an infant chair or swing while awake to help keep their nose clear. Laying down flat can also fill up the nose more.

- **TYLENOL®** – If your child has a fever and is irritable, TYLENOL® may be appropriate. Consult with your doctor.

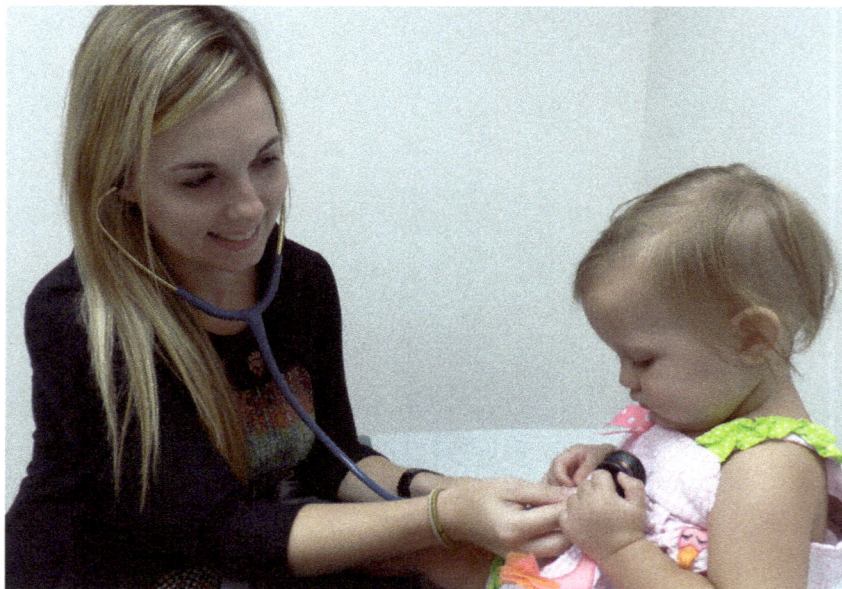

Ear Infections

Ear infections usually begin with a viral infection such as a cold. An ear infection is caused by fluid or mucus build-up in the middle ear. Symptoms to look for include ear pain, tugging or pulling at the ear, difficulty sleeping, unusual crying, irritability, loss of balance, fever over 100°F, drainage from the ear, loss of appetite, etc.

Croup

Croup causes a swelling of the voice box (larynx) and windpipe (trachea). Due to the swelling, the airway below the vocal cords becomes narrow and makes breathing difficult and noisy. Croup is most commonly due to an infection. It most often affects children between the ages of 3 months and 5 years. It can occur at any time but is most common in the fall and winter. The cough sounds like the bark of a seal.

If your child develops croup in the middle of the night, go into the bathroom and shut the door. Run the shower on the hottest setting and let the room steam up. This should help with his breathing within 15 to 20 minutes. The steam almost always works but if it does not, take him outside into the cool air. If your child is not improving, go to the nearest emergency room or call 911. If your child has croup, call our office in the morning for an appointment for evaluation.

Fever

If your child has a fever, that means he is fighting an infection. It is the body's normal response. There are several types of thermometers. For children under 4 or 5 years of age, you should take their temperature rectally.

Your child has a fever if he has a rectal or oral temperature over 100.4°F. If you cannot check the termperature orally, you should take it rectally. Ear and forehead temperatures can be inaccurate. Make sure your child is drinking plenty of liquids and he is wearing minimal clothing. Bundling him can cause a higher temperature.

If your child has a fever or seems uncomfortable, medication may be necessary. Follow the chart on the next page for medication dosage.

*If your child is under 2 months of age and has a fever he should go to the emergency room immediately. Do not give babies under the age of 3 months medication until speaking with your pediatrician.

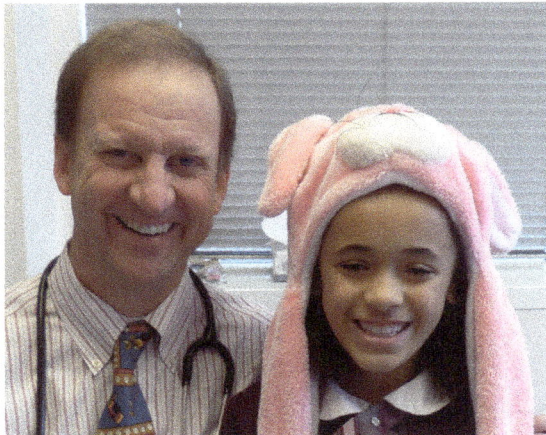

TYLENOL® (Acetaminophen)

Weight (lbs)	Age	Infants' TYLENOL® Oral Suspension (Acetaminophen 160 mg in each 5 mL)	Children's TYLENOL® Oral Suspension (Acetaminophen 160 mg in each 5 mL or 1 tsp)
6 – 11	0-3 Mths	1.25 mL	—
12 – 17	4-11 Mths	2.5 mL	—
18 – 23	12-23 Mths	3.75 mL	—
24 – 35	2-3 Yrs	5 mL	5 mL (1 tsp)

MOTRIN® (Ibuprofen)

Weight (lbs)	Age	Infants' MOTRIN® Oral Suspension (Ibuprofen 100 mg in each 5 mL)	Children's MOTRIN® Oral Suspension (Ibuprofen 100 mg in each 5 mL or 1 tsp)
6 – 11	0-5 Mths	Do Not Use	—
12 – 17	6-11 Mths	1.25 mL	—
18 – 23	12-23 Mths	1.875 mL	—
24 – 35	2-3 Yrs	—	5 mL (1 tsp)

*For both TYLENOL® and MOTRIN®, If possible, use weight to dose; otherwise use age.

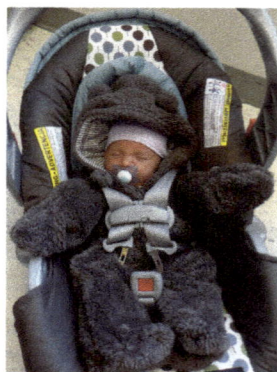

Vaccines

We strongly recommend infants and children receive their vaccines on the following schedule. The vaccines are timed in order to protect your child when his is most vulnerable and when they will be most effective. Vaccines do not cause autism nor will they "overwhelm" your child's immune system. The American Academy of Pediatrics has an excellent website at **www.aap.org** that can answer any questions you have. Vaccines protect your child against life threatening disease. Feel free to ask any of our providers about vaccine questions you have.

Regular Immunization Schedule

Age	Vaccine
1 Month	Hep B #2
2 Month	DTAP #1, IPV #1, PCV #1, HIB #1, ROTA #1
4 Month	DTAP #2, IPV #2, PCV #2, HIB #2, ROTA #2
6 Month	DTAP #3, PCV #3, HIB #3, ROTA #3
9 Month	HEP B #3
12 Month	VAR #1, PCV #4, HIB #4
15 Month	MMR #1, HEP A #1
18 Month	DTAP #4, IPV #3
2 Year	HEP A #2
3 Year	None
4 Year	MMR #2, VAR #2
5 Year	DTAP #5, IPV #4

Annual flu vaccines are recommended. Children will receive 2 doses the first year (1st dose after 6 months of age) and then 1 dose each year thereafter.

Explanation of abbreviated vaccines above:

IPV:	Polio		**VAR:**	Chicken Pox
PCV:	Prevnar		**MMR:**	Measles/Mumps/Rubella
DTAP:	Diphtheria/tetanus/pertussis		**HEPB:**	Hepatitis B
ROTA:	Rotavirus Vaccine - oral		**HEPA:**	Hepatitis A
HIB:	Haemophilus Influenzae B			

This immunization schedule is subject to change.

Safety

Car Seats

It's very important to read the manual of your car seat to make sure it is installed correctly. The seat should be snug to the rear seat and not move more than 1 inch from side to side. Follow the chart below for optimal safety.

Age Group	Type of Seat	General Guidelines
Infants/Toddlers	Rear-facing only seats and rear-facing convertible seats	All infants and toddlers should ride in a **Rear-Facing Car Seat** until they reach the highest weight or height allowed by their car seat's manufacturer.
Toddlers/Preschoolers	Convertible seats and forward-facing seats with harnesses	All children who have outgrown the rearfacing car seat should use a **Forward-Facing Car Seat** with a harness for as long as possible, up to the highest weight or height allowed by their car seat manufacturer.
School-Aged Children	Booster seats	All children who have outgrown the forwardfacing car seat should use a **Booster Seat** until the vehicle seat belt fits properly.

For more information on child safety seats, visit **www.nhtsa.gov**. A certified child passenger safety technician can check your installation and answer any questions. To locate one near you, visit **www.seatcheck.org**.

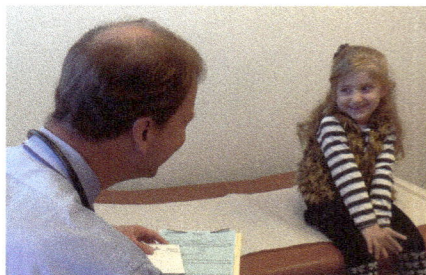

Choking

A choking child is a very scary event. Your baby can choke on anything he puts into his mouth. Be aware of any objects around that your baby could possibly put in his mouth. Keep items that are choking hazards away from your child.

These include:

- Coins
- Buttons
- Toys with small parts
- Toys that can fit entirely in a child's mouth
- Small balls and marbles

- Balloons
- Small hair bows, barrettes, and rubber bands
- Pen or marker caps
- Small button-type batteries
- Refrigerator magnets

Certain foods are more of a choking hazard than others. Be sure to cut your child's food into pieces no larger than ½ inch. When your child is eating, he should be sitting and not moving around a lot. Keep the following foods away from children under the age of 4:

- Hot dogs
- Nuts and seeds
- Chunks of meat or cheese
- Whole grapes
- Hard or sticky candy

- Popcorn
- Chunks of peanut butter
- Chunks of raw vegetables
- Chewing gum

It is recommended that all parents take a CPR class to learn how to properly help a child or adult when they are choking.

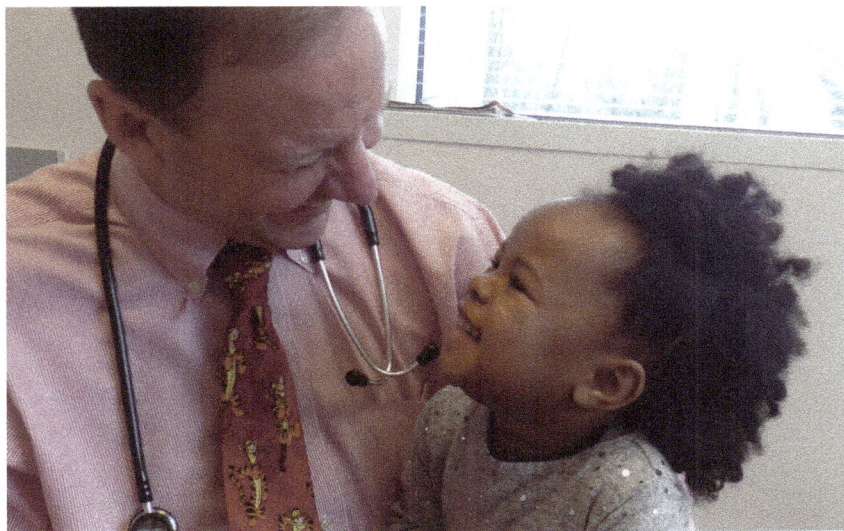

Healthcare Record

1 to 2 Week Visit

Date:_____ **Wt:**_____ **Ht:**_____ **HC:**_____

Diet: Formula or breast milk.

Development: Hearing is fully developed, eyes focus well at about 12" from face. Yawns, sneezes and hiccups. Startles to noise, has interest in the human voice.

Socialization: Try to establish eye contact with your baby. Give brightly colored toys, like a mobile. Talk to your baby, smile at him and enjoy him.

Notes:_____

_____

_____

_____

_____

_____

_____

1 Month Visit

Date:_____ **Wt:**_____ **Ht:**_____ **HC:**_____

Diet: Formula or breast milk.

Development: Starts to smile, raises head when on tummy, settles down when rocked, held and sung to.

Socialization: Cuddle your baby and sing to him, letting him know you're there.

Notes:_____

_____

_____

_____

_____

_____

_____

2 Month Visit

Date:_____ Wt:_____ Ht:_____ HC:_____

Diet: Formula or breast milk.

Development: Recognizes his caregiver. Smiles at people and begins to coo and make other noises. He may start sleeping through the night.

Socialization: Smile back at your baby. Place different textures and toys in his hands, like a musical toy.

Notes:_____

_____

_____

_____

_____

_____

_____

4 Month Visit

Date:_____ Wt:_____ Ht:_____ HC:_____

Diet: Formula or breast milk.

Development: Lifts his head and upper body off the ground when lying on his stomach. He may be rolling over and will look around when someone enters the room or calls his name. Giggles when tickled and babbles.

Socialization: Give your baby grasping toys or toys to bat at. Child mirrors are a great toy for this age. Introduce the game pat-a-cake.

Notes:_____

_____

_____

_____

_____

_____

_____

6 Month Visit

Date:_____ **Wt:**_____ **Ht:**_____ **HC:**_____

Diet: Formula or breast milk. Solid food is not necessary but you can introduce fruit and vegetables. We suggest introducing vegetables, then fruits. Allow a few days between the introduction of each new food to watch for signs of food allergy, such as diarrhea or a rash.

Development: May sit well alone, or with some support. Expresses definite emotions such as fear, anger and loneliness. Teeth may appear, usually the lower ones. Helps hold his bottle and puts everything in his mouth.

Socialization: Play "peek-a-boo" with your baby.

Notes:_____
_____
_____
_____
_____
_____
_____

9 Month Visit

Date:_____ **Wt:**_____ **Ht:**_____ **HC:**_____

Diet: Formula or breast milk, pureed meat, fruits and vegetables. Introduce a sippy cup.

Development: Sits well and may try to stand or walk holding onto furniture. Can pick up a small object using two fingers. Understands specific commands, such as "no" and may say "ma-ma" or "da-da".

Socialization: Let your baby hold your hands and try to walk. Introduce toys with different shapes and sounds. Point out familiar objects and repeat their names.

Notes:_____
_____
_____
_____
_____
_____
_____

12 Month Visit

Date:_____ **Wt:**_____ **Ht:**_____ **HC:**_____

Diet: Wean off the bottle and start whole milk. You may continue breastfeeding. For most children, no water or juice regularly until 2 years old.

Development: Walks with support or may take steps alone, picks up small objects and eats with his fingers. He may say one to three meaningful words besides "mama" and "da-da". He waves bye-bye and claps hands. Cries when mom or dad leaves.

Socialization: Encourage social games such as peek-a-boo and pat-a-cake. Encourage speech development by naming common objects and point out body parts.

Notes:_____

_____

_____

_____

_____

_____

_____

15 Month Visit

Date:_____ **Wt:**_____ **Ht:**_____ **HC:**_____

Diet: Your baby may exhibit strong food preferences. Remember that children of this age typically do not eat much and commonly are "picky eaters".

Development: Walks independently with confidence, and may even run and climb. Your child uses utensils at mealtime, and can point to a few body parts. Drinks from a cup.

Socialization: Encourage imitative behaviors with pretend play such as cooking, cleaning, working with tools and driving.

Notes:_____

Notes:_____

_____

_____

_____

_____

_____

_____

18 Month Visit

Date:_____ **Wt:**_____ **Ht:**_____ **HC:**_____

Diet: Your child will be very opinionated with what he wants. Try to avoid struggles at mealtime.

Development: Climbs stairs while holding the railing or your hand. He kicks and throws balls. His vocabulary may consist of about 10 words, and he may begin to combine two-word phrases.

Socialization: Encourage your child's curiosity independence.

Notes:_____
_____
_____
_____
_____
_____
_____

2 Year Visit

Date:_____ **Wt:**_____ **Ht:**_____ **HC:**_____

Diet: Your child will continue to be very opinionated with what he wants.

Development: Names many familiar things. Is able to entertain himself while playing alone and also plays well with an adult. Can point to several body parts when asked and starts to undress himself. Turns book pages one at a time.

Socialization: Encourage your child's curiosity and interest in learning new things like songs, letters, etc. Also, nurture his independence.

Notes:_____
_____
_____
_____
_____
_____
_____

Resources

Important Numbers

Poison Control. **1.800.222.1222**

Children's Healthcare of Atlanta/Scottish Rite **404.785.5252**

Children's Healthcare of Atlanta/Egleston **404.785-6000**

Breastfeeding and Newborn Resources

Breastfeeding Made Simple: Seven Natural Laws for Nursing Mothers by Nancy Mohrbacher, IBCLC FILCA & Kathleen Kendall-Tackett PhD IBCLC (December 1, 2010)

The Breastfeeding Mother's Guide to Making More Milk: Foreward by Martha Sears, RN by Diana West and Lisa Marasco

The Happiest Baby on the Block by Harvey Karp

On Becoming Baby Wise by Gary Ezzo and Robert Buckman

Le Leche League: www.lllofga.org

Medela: www.medelabreastfeedingus.com

Strong4life.com

Loveandlogic.com

Trustworthy Websites

American Academy of Pediatrics . . . . www.aap.org

Healthy Children. . . . . www.healthychildren.org

Centers for Disease Control. . . . . www.cdc.org

Food Allergy Research & Educations . . . . www.foodallergy.org

Recommended Reading

1. **Heading Home With Your Newborn: Birth To Reality**, Laura Jana, M.D., FAAP and Jennifer Shu, M.D., FAAP

2. **Caring for Your Baby and Young Child Birth to Age 5**, by Dr. Steven P. Shelov for the American Academy of Pediatrics

3. HealthyChildren.org

Notes

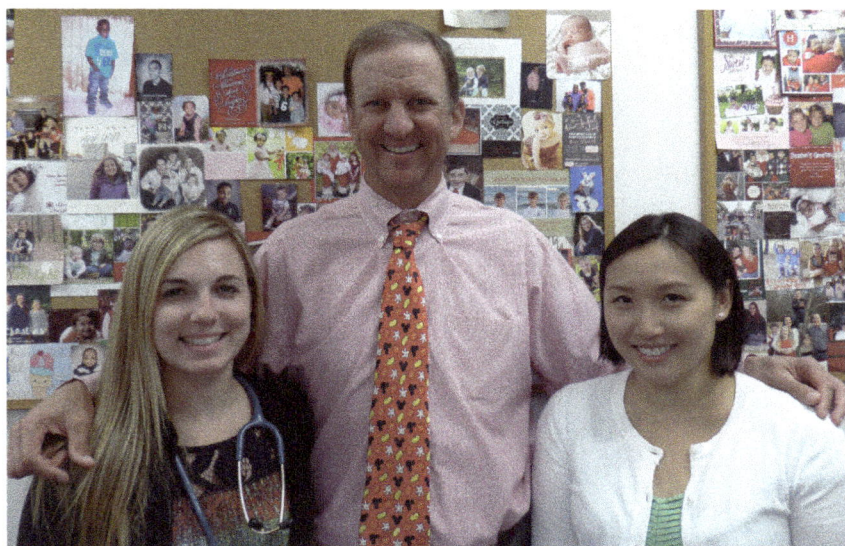

Putting CARE back in HealthCare

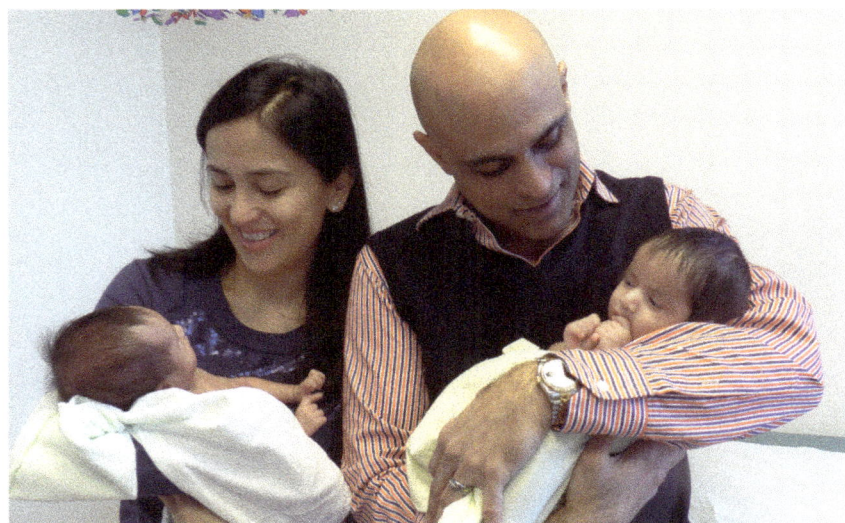

Our Physicians

John M. Thomas, Jr., M.D.

Dr. Thomas has lived in Atlanta since 1978. He attended college at the University of Georgia, attended medical school at The Medical College of Georgia and completed his residency at Kosair Children's Hospital of Louisville. "I have always believed in treating each patient the way I would care for my own child" is Dr. Thomas' philosophy. Dr. Thomas enjoys family, golf and scuba diving.

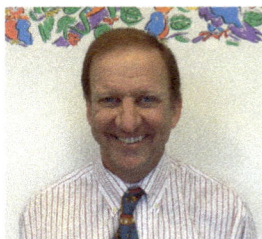

Willa F. Moore, M.D.

Dr. Moore grew up in Shaker Heights, Ohio. Board certified in Pediatrics, Dr. Moore received her medical degree from Northeast Ohio Medical University, her internship and residency in Pediatrics at University Hospitals Rainbow Babies & Children's Hospital in Cleveland, Ohio. Early in her training, she gravitated toward pediatrics because it is a specialty that allows physicians to develop continuing relationships with patients and families. In her spare time, she enjoys traveling, cooking, and spending time outdoors with her husband and dog.

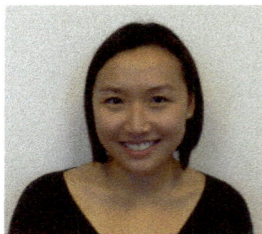

Jessica E. Norris, M.D.

Jessica grew up in Suwanee, GA with her parents, older brother and older sister. She graduated with a Degree in Biology from the University of GA in 2008 and with her MD in 2012 from the Medical College of Ga in Augusta. She then went on to St. Louis for three years to complete her pediatric residency. She loves spending time with her family, her black lab "Champ" and cheering on her favorite football team, the GA Bulldogs, with her dad. She is excited to move back closer to family and start taking care of patients at Children's Care!

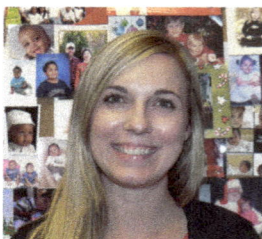

Index